CONGRATULATIONS! By opening this book, you've accomplished the first step in achieving a successful body transformation: the DESIRE to change. Whether you want to lose fifty pounds or five, without this first step you will never get there. It is the only step that you have to do completely on your own, and often times it is the most difficult. Now that you've conquered the first step of the process on your own, it is time to find some help with the rest. We wrote this book to help get you through the rest of those steps on your fat loss journey.

In this book, you will find fifty-two different ways to burn body fat more efficiently, separated into four distinctly different categories. However, trying to do ALL of these tips at once can lead to information overload, resulting in you ending up more confused than when you started! That is why we designed it so that you can pull ONE tip from the book each week and just master that technique before moving onto another one. You see, it is the MASTERY of these simple fat loss strategies that lead to long term success, not the IMPLEMENTATION alone. Simply doing everything once will not get you to your fat loss goals. It takes repetition to turn these tips into habits. If you are able to master one technique each week, before moving onto the next, by the end of the year you will have created fifty-two daily habits that are now second nature to you! If you can accomplish that, your fat loss results will be better than you could have ever imagined before you started reading this book!

Start off by browsing though the book and see which of these strategies sound familiar. Remember, these guidelines are not "secrets". Chances are that some of these tips are things that you have already built into your daily or weekly routine. If you can check those ones off as MASTERED, not "oh, occasionally I do that," then you are a step closer to reaching all fifty-two, and therefore, a step ahead in achieving your fat loss goals. After you have identified which ones you have already mastered, begin by choosing the new fat loss technique that you have the highest chance of completing and STICKING to that first week. It is SO important that you get off on the right foot and find success with the first couple strategies that you choose in order to get positive momentum. Over the course of the year (and further on down the road), it is consistency that will give you the best results as opposed to peaks of adherence followed by valleys of regression.

Hopefully you will find this book useful in achieving your goals and the methods enclosed to be valuable additions to your daily life. Remember that there is NO failure when undertaking a positive life change such as this, and also no finish line. Enjoy the process. Every day is a new opportunity to create a

successful habit. Hopefully, in a year's time, you will have fifty-two new ones, and a body transformation that you can be proud of!

<u>IMPORTANT</u>:

Consult with your physician before beginning any diet or exercise program, including the tips found in this book. We do not accept responsibility for any injuries obtained using the techniques we outline, so please always use the help of a qualified professional.

__Lifestyle__

The fat loss tips found in this category have little to do with exercise and nutrition, and more to do with incorporating healthy habits into your life that will help you burn extra calories with little change to your daily routine. Many of these tips are very small changes and are sometimes the easiest to implement and stick to, making it a good place to start.

Find PHYSICAL Activities That You Enjoy Doing

Notice how the word PHYSICAL is capitalized? It is to make sure you know how important it is to be active in order to burn fat. Most people spend large portions of their day sitting at work, burning very few calories. When it's time to unwind with some down time, do not spend it on the couch watching re-runs on the T.V. Get up and be active! Experiment with different physical activities until you find one (or many) that you really LIKE doing. It could be something as easy as hiking, tennis, ping-pong, or just going for a walk. They do not have to be sports. They do not have to be exhausting, but they should require you to get up and move that body of yours around for a bit. Start with a small goal of fifteen minutes and increase the duration from there.

Take the Stairs

When you are working, there may not be many opportunities to sneak in some physical activity. One way is to skip the elevator and use the stairs whenever you have to go to a different floor. If you have not walked a couple flights of stairs in a while, you might be surprised at the difficulty of such a seemingly simple task. Start slow if need be and only take them when you have to go up one floor. Then, graduate to two flights and three and so on. If you are reading this in your skyscraper office, resist the urge to climb every step in your building. Just start with a few floors at a time.

Get an Ergonomic Workstation

Even though having your chair, computer, mouse, etc. set up perfectly to fit your body will not actually burn any additional calories, it WILL help you look and feel better, increasing your ability to perform more physical activity down the road. If you are always slouching, or your shoulders and back hurt from hunching over a computer all day, what is the likelihood that you will leave work and hit the gym for a workout? When your body feels good, you want to use it! Talk to your supervisor about getting your desk set up properly A.S.A.P. Mention how much more productive it will make you at work, and they will quickly comply!

Stretch at Work

Much like having an ergonomic workspace will not directly burn more calories, the benefits of taking some time to stretch while at work will pay off greatly over time. First, it requires you to actually get up and move away from your workspace, which is something far too few people do during the average workday. Second, stretching out tense muscles that get tight and sore over the course of the day from overuse (muscles in the neck and lower back are frequently strained due to hunching over a computer keyboard all day) can reduce the risk of longer term problems with these areas. This can prevent you from missing workouts due to sore muscles. Third, an increase in overall flexibility leads to the ability to perform a larger amount of physical activities without the risk of injury, expanding your exercise library.

Park Farther Away

How many times have you gone to the mall or grocery store and seen that person driving up and down the aisles looking for that perfect parking spot? Perhaps you have been guilty of it yourself from time-to-time. An easy way to burn a few extra calories each day (and save some time as well) is to just take that first available spot, even if it is a few extra yards. It does not have to be the farthest available spot in the lot. A few extra yards will add up over time. You could do this at work, the store, picking up kids at school, anywhere. If you add one hundred extra yards per day to your daily walking total from parking alone, you will walk nearly a half a mile extra each week. Over the course of a year, it will be nearly an entire marathon!

Chew Gum

The simple act of chewing gum burns a whopping eleven calories per hour. Additionally, it increases your metabolism, and by doing so, this becomes quite an effective fat burning strategy. The act of chewing alone can trick your body into thinking it is consuming food, and help curb appetite, especially for sweets. Make sure to get a low sugar gum, and one without artificial sweeteners (such as aspartame) in it.

Suck In Your Gut

One of the most underdeveloped muscles in the human body today is the transverse abdominus, the abdominal muscles responsible for keeping the "core" tight. Because of the high amount of sitting and the overemphasis on crunches, this muscle often gets overlooked. However, it is the muscle most responsible for keeping a tight stomach, which we all want. By sucking in your gut throughout the day, you are actually strengthening those muscles that hold everything in place. Try tying a string around your waist so that when you relax your abdominals, you feel a mild discomfort. This method not only trains your stomach to be pulled in more naturally, but helps increase the strength and endurance of the muscles stabilizing the spine, preventing future lower back injuries due to weakness of the "core".

Moderate Alcohol Consumption

Chances are, you are not interested in giving up drinking permanently. That is okay! However, you should try to limit the amounts that you drink. The body can only do so many things at one time. Eliminating alcohol from your system and fat burning are two that cannot be done together. For every hour that your body spends processing the drinks you had at happy hour last night equals the amount of hours it was unable to burn fat. In addition, many alcohols make the claim that they are low calorie or calorie free, but they are not required to disclose the amount of "sugar alcohols" in the product, which contain 7 calories per gram. These calories can add up pretty quick, especially if you are mixing it with sugar laden beverages for taste.

<u>Create Habits or Rituals</u>

Most people have a set of daily habits that they perform and have done so for years. Even the most disorganized person has things that they do strictly out of routine. One of the difficulties of fat loss is that it requires the formation of NEW habits, ones that are often times the complete opposite of the person's normal routine. With some willpower, you can turn new responsibilities (like packing your lunch and prepping your food) into a new and improved daily routine. It has been said that it takes three weeks for something to become a habit. If you can stick it out that long, chances are that you will be able to maintain the new healthier habit long term. Remember, every daily ritual you already have took some time to become a habit. At some point in your life, you had to set aside an extra couple of minutes each morning and night to brush your teeth. I am certain you would not skip that routine now would you? These new habits are no different!

Get a Good Night's Sleep

For some, sleeping seems like a waste of time. Something that we HAVE to do for a few hours, but sleep is probably the most important part of our day. Without it, we would not be able to function properly. Have you ever woken up from a poor night's sleep and felt sluggish the rest of the day? Most people have. Conversely, have you woken up from a good night's sleep and felt super refreshed and energized? It makes quite the difference! The amount of things that you can achieve on a day after good sleep (such as exercising and being productive) are far greater than after a poor night of shut eye. The recommended amount of time to sleep has been shown to be about seven to nine hours on average. Most people sleep less than that. If you are one of those and you think that you get by just fine on six hours or less, chances are that you do not remember what it feels like to wake from a really good sleep! You can train your mind to grow accustomed to how you feel after waking up after five to six hours every day, but you CANNOT train your brain to do everything it needs to do in five hours of sleep instead of eight.

Bring Snacks With You on the Road

Employing this habit can save you THOUSANDS of empty calories each week. Think about the places you go where it has become a tradition to eat unhealthy foods that derail your fat loss goals. These can include family dinners, office potlucks, and movie theaters. Unfortunately, all of these place an emphasis on consuming high fat, high carbohydrate, high sugar foods. It can be extremely tempting to indulge in these foods when placed directly in front of you. The solution: bring your own healthier snacks to these types of events. Try bringing a healthy entrée to dinner, a veggie plate to the potluck, or even your own fresh popped popcorn to the movies. Having these types of food on hand can help you circumvent some of the dietary pitfalls that plague even the most diligent of dieters.

<u>Simplify Your Life</u>

Instead of trying to master the minutia, try to focus on the absolute basics of good health, and MASTER them! A couple of the basic principles of fat loss, turned into daily habits, will provide MUCH greater results than many little things done sporadically over time. Too often people become concerned with things like "What is the perfect carbohydrate source two hours before I workout if I'm training legs on a Wednesday afternoon." Then that same person has french fries the next day for lunch. Do not over analyze what you need to do to achieve your goals. Nobody eats 100% clean and has A+ workouts all the time, so do not chase the perfect week. Aim to change one thing at a time and eventually you will have mastered several important new habits that will have you on the fast track to success.

EXERCISE

We all know that we need to exercise in order to keep our bodies healthy, but that doesn't mean that you need to spend hours upon hours each day on the treadmill in order to burn that unwanted fat. Simply try these exercise tips to make your workouts more productive, leaving you more time to enjoy the rest of your life!

HIIT Training

Otherwise known as High Intensity Interval Training, HIIT training alternates bouts of short, intense exercise with less intense recovery periods. This type of training increases aerobic capacity (your body's ability to utilize oxygen). It also leads to a greater calorie burn up to 36 hours post workout due to the excess post exercise oxygen consumption (EPOC). What does this mean for you? You burn more calories even when your workout is over, AND you can exercise for shorter durations.

Use Your Bodyweight

Moving your body is the easiest way to get in a workout. You already have the equipment, it is YOU! Doing callisthenic exercises such as jumping jacks, pushups, bodyweight rows, and squats can build muscle and burn fat, without having to go to the gym. What does it mean for you? This means you have the convenience of being able to work out anytime, anywhere.

__Periodization__

Most people go into the gym and think, "What should I do today?" The BEST results in the gym come from having a plan that is structured and gets increasingly more difficult over time. As the body adapts to exercise, it requires greater demands to be placed on it in order to continue to progress. Have a plan in place so that when you go to the gym, you know your workout will be a little bit harder than last time.

<u>Lift Heavy</u>

"I thought we were talking about fat loss? I don't want big muscles!" Do not worry, we will not be bulking up in this training tip. Lifting heavy weights has benefits for everyone, such as enhanced muscle tone and higher post workout calorie burn. "Heavy weights" is a relative term. It is not a standard number for everyone, but rather a range of repetitions that proves to be difficult to complete for each individual person, approximately eight to twelve per set. Lifting weights in this zone will provide a stimulus to build muscle, thereby increasing fat loss down the road.

Fasted Cardio

Doing your cardiovascular training first thing in the morning on an empty stomach has proven to be an effective method for burning fat, especially those last few pounds of stubborn body fat that NEVER seem to come off. The reason? When you wake in the morning, your liver glycogen stores are very near empty because you have been "fasting" as you sleep. This forces your body to turn to an alternative source of fuel for the exercise, FAT. The result is that you use more of your fat stores to fuel your workout as opposed to doing it after breakfast. **Note**: If you have not tried this before, keep the workout intensity fairly low at the beginning to avoid feeling sick. Even a short duration walk first thing in the morning will be beneficial.

Something Is Better Than Nothing

All too often people will take the "all or nothing" approach when it comes to working out. They have to have all the stars aligned to have the absolute best workout they could imagine. More often than not, this leads to more missed workouts than amazing ones. The solution? Do not be dissatisfied with doing just a little bit. A lot of little workouts add up to big results. If you forgot your workout clothes, go for a walk. If your knee hurts, do some upper body training. Do something. You'll not only feel better because you did not miss a workout, but you will keep the habit of continuing to work out in place by not missing it entirely.

Do Compound Exercises

A compound exercise is a lift that requires the use of many different muscles at the same time. These would include squats, deadlifts, lunges, step ups, bench press, shoulder press, rowing and pulldown movements. These exercises build muscle quickly, and burn more calories than other exercises due to the amount of muscles involved in the lift. A bicep curl works just the biceps. A row, on the other hand, works the biceps as well as the rhomboids, trapezius, and latissimus dorsi among others. If you are looking for fat loss, these compound exercises must become the staple of your routines.

Spend Less Time On "Abs"

As counterintuitive as that sounds, training your abs via exercises such as crunches and leg raises does little to actually burn fat. The abdominal muscles that make up the "six pack" are fairly small, and therefore, do not require large amounts of energy (or calories) to work them. They also do not build as easily as other muscle groups, and thus, have a limited effect on increasing metabolism. Instead of devoting 15 minutes to abs at the end of your workouts, use that time to do some of the compound movements discussed earlier like squats, rows, and pushups.

Use Supersets, Tri-sets, and Giant sets

A superset is two different exercises performed back to back, a tri set is three and a giant set is four or more. Structuring your workout to include these will help you get more done in less time, raise your heart rate throughout your workout, and get you through your workout faster. Pair up exercises that work the same muscle group, such as a triceps pressdown with a bench dip. You can also work opposing muscle groups such as back and chest or quads and hamstrings. Alternating between upper and lower body exercises will increase your fat burn even higher, as your heart rate has to climb to meet the demand of pumping blood to the muscles of both the upper and lower limbs. Instead of resting between sets of squats, drop down and do some pushups to incinerate more fat.

Slow It Down

Most people will rush through their reps as fast as they can in order to finish a particular exercise. By slowing down the movements, especially the eccentric (or lowering) phase of the movement, you can increase the time under tension of the target muscles, thus making them work harder and burn more calories. Give it a try on your next workout. You will find that the sets are more difficult to complete with your normal weights, and you will notice a new muscle soreness from the increased muscular tension!

<u>Listen To Your Favorite Music</u>

Studies show that people who listen to their favorite upbeat music tend to workout harder and longer than those who do not. You should not rely on the soundtrack playing over the speakers at your local gym. Get your iPod or phone and create a specific playlist or mix that will fire you up to workout! Make sure that you keep the slow jams off the list. You want to choose tunes that inspire you and motivate you to work hard and keep up the pace. Try it out! It could be the difference between an average workout and a great one!

<u>PSYCHOLOGICAL</u>

The tips in this section of the book are included specifically to help you conquer the mental challenges of trying to lose weight. We have taken some of the most common pitfalls experienced by our own clients over the last decade and designed specific strategies to avoid or overcome them. These tips will help keep you motivated, on track, and accountable over the long term pursuit of your goals.

Weigh In Weekly

We live in a world of instant gratification where we want things as quickly as possible. When it comes to losing weight and burning fat, we are no different. We step on the scale every day, hoping that the salad we ate for lunch yesterday made us lose that extra pound. However, losing body fat is a little more complicated than that. It is not an instantaneous process. If it was, we would not need to write this book! Fat loss occurs over a series of changes in the body and takes longer than a day to materialize. Save yourself the anguish of weighing in every day and try to do it once a week on a specific day, at a specific time. The most accurate time is right after waking and going to the bathroom because this will give you the most consistent results.

Take Bodyfat Measurements

Do not rely only on the scale when your goal is to lose BODYFAT. Scales tell you weight, and that is it. Sometimes when you are on a fat loss journey, you can reach a plateau on the scale. This does not necessarily mean you aren't burning fat still. Sometimes you build more muscle on a given week, or you drank more water. Use a device that measures how much of your weight is muscle, water, and fat. Simple handheld calipers can be found at most gyms and use a mathematic formula to determine an estimated bodyfat level. You could also use calipers that measure skin folds, but these usually require a skilled professional in order to get an accurate, consistent result. Whichever method you choose, be consistent and perform it weekly like you would with your weigh-ins.

Use Before and After Pictures

Often times people will be motivated to lose weight as a result of seeing an old picture of themselves when they were in better shape, or a new photograph where they realize that they are out of shape. The reason? Most people respond more favorably to visual stimulus. You can use this to your advantage by either finding an old photograph of yourself you want to look like, or a photo that you never want to look like again. Whichever one you choose is up to you depending on what motivates you. Either way, we recommend documenting your progress through pictures taken throughout your fat loss efforts so that you can VISUALLY see the results, and not solely rely on the numbers on the scale.

Schedule Your Workouts In A Calendar

Having your workouts set up in your Outlook, iMac, or whatever you use to organize your day, is a great way to make sure you make the time to do it. Treat it as if it is just another appointment in your book, something that you are required to do. This will help to create the habit of getting to the gym without allowing things to get in the way of your "appointment."

Write Short and Long Term Goals

Many times, people have a vision of their ideal self, and they set a lofty goal with a big weight loss number. The problem is that they have no idea how to get there! What steps are you going to take to reach your ultimate long term goal? These small daily, weekly, and monthly ACTION goals are what create success. Action goals detail exactly what you will do in order to help you achieve your goal. A daily action goal is to drink at least 8 cups of water. A weekly action goal is to avoid eating takeout for the week. These are the actions that you will take to reach your long term goal. Without them, you will not have a defined path on how to get there.

Tell People About Your Goals

When people share a goal or a task they are undertaking with others (friends, family, or even through social media), they are much more likely to achieve that goal. The idea of letting others down is a very powerful motivator, and you are more likely to stick it out when the going gets tough, knowing that others are going to hold you accountable.

<u>Find YOUR Motivation</u>

Every person's motivation is different. You have to find YOURS! And trust me, it is NOT a number on a scale. This is an example of an extrinsic motivator. This type of motivation is good, but is not nearly as powerful as intrinsic motivators. These would include getting in shape to play with your kids, or preventing the onset of disease in your family history. Whatever it is that motivates you the most, FIND IT! The deeper the motivation, the more you will be inclined not to fail.

Surround Yourself with Positive People

When you are trying to lose fat, it helps to associate with people who are attempting to do the same thing. This way, you are able to feed off of each other's success and also keep each other accountable. Even if your friends/family do not have the same goals as you, they still can be supportive of your efforts. If you have a coworker who likes to go out to lunch every day and eat unhealthy foods, then you need to distance yourself from that person in order to stay on track. It may seem a bit selfish, but it will affect your motivation level. If you have the right motivation, a takeout lunch probably will not seem as appealing.

Stick With It

We have more information than ever at our disposal today. The internet allows us to find thousands of exercise and nutrition tips and strategies that may or may not work. Often times, we are trying multiple things at once in order to try and speed up our results. However, sometimes these different strategies do not work synergistically with each other. Doing one program simultaneously with another can actually slow down your fat loss efforts. The way to combat this is to pick ONE method and stick with it for a specific length of time. Then, analyze your results with the program and if it is working, keep doing it! If it did not meet your expectations, move onto a different program and give that your undivided attention. This way, you know if each individual diet or workout regimen is working for YOU. Note: Give a program at least four weeks of honest effort before assessing whether to move on or not.

Find a Workout Buddy

Having someone there with the same goal as you can provide the extra motivation you need to stay on track. Whether they make you go to the gym on one of those days when you just feel like skipping, or they suggest a healthy restaurant instead of takeout, having that person there on your fat loss journey can be the difference between success and failure.

Try a Group Exercise Class

One of the hottest new trends in the fitness industry today is the gravitation towards group exercise. Programs like CrossFit, bootcamps, and spin classes are getting increasingly high attendance rates and adherence rates. Why? Because these types of activities are creating COMMUNITIES amongst their members. People working together as a group are stronger than someone working alone. Members of these types of classes are feeding off each other, and getting better results because of it! When looking to join a group exercise class, it is important to look for something that is congruent with the goals you want to achieve, and that the people within the group are somewhat like yourself. These two things will make the overall experience a much more pleasant and successful one.

<u>NUTRITION:</u>

We saved this section of the book for last because it is the MOST important factor in fat loss, and we want these tips to be fresh in your mind as you finish the book. Do not underestimate the importance of your nutrition in reaching your goals. All of the strategies in this book cannot overcome an unhealthy diet. That being said, it is entirely possible to enjoy the food you eat and still lose weight. Changing a few dietary habits here and there can make all the difference in the world when it comes to fat loss.

<u>Eat More Protein</u>

Increasing the amount of protein in your diet has many benefits. It will help aid in the repair/building of muscle tissue. It will help you feel more full after meals because of the energy it takes to chew and digest it. It acts as a thermogenic during the digestion process, burning more calories than other macronutrients. There are many varieties of protein to choose from, including lean beef, pork, chicken, fish, turkey, eggs, dairy products, and shellfish. Your body needs the essential amino acids found in these protein sources in order to complete many everyday functions, including burning fat. Grab a fork and knife and eat your protein! About a gram per kilogram of bodyweight every day is a good place to start.

Consume Healthy Fats

"If I am trying to lose fat, why would I eat it?" Well, the human body needs HEALTHY fats to survive. They provide benefits such as increased brain function, improved eyesight, proper energy metabolism, and more. They also help the absorption of fat-soluble vitamins and minerals. Now you should not just eat any fats, there are certain types that are better than others. Healthy fats include olive and vegetable oils, avocados, nuts and seeds, and coconut oil (a must have for every kitchen). Be careful on the serving size when you eat your healthy fats, because they are more calorie dense than both protein and carbohydrate. One tablespoon contains about twelve grams of fat, which is over a hundred calories. Make sure to avoid processed fats such as trans fats at all costs. These types of fat contain no nutritional value and have been shown to cause serious health problems when consumed over time. These can be found in products with long shelf lives, such as cookies, crackers, and other snack foods.

Moderate Carbohydrate Intake

The typical American diet tends to lean very heavily on "carbs" as the primary source of fuel for our bodies. The FDA recommends 300 carbohydrates a day for the average person. The food pyramid puts grains as the primary food source on the pyramid. The problem with that is that most of the carbohydrates we consume come from *manufactured* sources, foods that are processed and have long shelf lives. These are typically convenience foods and include chemicals and un-pronounceable ingredients. The trade off for cheap, easy manufacturing is that the ingredients in these foods can cause quick weight gain. Stick to the more natural sources of carbohydrates, such as fruits, veggies, oatmeal, brown rice, quinoa, and legumes. Leave the processed stuff on the shelves.

Stay On the Perimeter of the Grocery Store

Consider what you have learned about ways to improve our nutrition and apply it directly to your grocery shopping experience. Stay on the perimeter of the grocery store, which will keep you in the sections that contain the types of foods you want to eat. Here you will find lean meats, fruits, veggies, healthy dairy products, eggs, and nuts. What you will not find is boxed items, canned foods, or other processed foods. The foods on the perimeter should make up the bulk of your daily nutrition plan.

<u>Make a Plan</u>

Planning is a crucial step in any fat loss program, and would be listed number one importance in this section, if I was listing them by rank. "Without a plan is planning to fail." This quote rings especially true when it comes to eating for fat loss. You must have a plan or eating schedule in place, along with the proper meals and snacks available to you at all times throughout the day. Otherwise, you will deviate from your goal of eating healthy. Most people eat because they are "hungry;" their body is sending them signals that it needs food quickly. The result? Reaching for whatever is most convenient in order to satisfy that hunger. This is the most challenging foe on our fat loss journey, and often claims even the most dedicated of healthy eaters. In order to avoid the hunger pains and temptation to cheat, make sure to plan ahead and have your healthy snacks ready.

Prepare Your Meals in Bulk

One of the problems people run into when it comes to maintaining a healthy eating lifestyle is the time it takes to prepare all of their food. Let's face it, it takes longer than getting it out of a box, but that does not mean you should abandon the cause, nor spend every second of free time cooking food. The solution is to multi task and make a few meals at once. Do not prepare a single serving of chicken breast seven days a week. Throw seven chicken breasts on the grill and then put the six you do not eat in a Tupperware container for the next day. While making breakfast, throw some ingredients in the crockpot and you will have dinner ready for you when you get home. If you are making a nice fancy dinner, make some extra and take the leftovers for lunch the next day. Be creative and you will spend less time in the kitchen than you think.

Make Adjustments to Your Diet Periodically

The human body is an incredibly efficient machine. Its primary goal is to use as little energy as possible in order to complete its daily functions, and then conserve the rest as a survival mechanism against starvation. The problem is that we as a species are no longer faced with long periods of famine and drought, and many of us have food available to us every day. After a period of calorie restriction, the body can adapt to a lower amount of calories and start storing body fat again. In order to prevent this, adjust the quantities of the calories on a daily or weekly basis, fooling the body's fat storing mechanisms into continuing to burn excess body fat for fuel. This technique is called calorie cycling, and can help eliminate the dreaded plateau that most dieters inevitably hit.

Use a Calorie Count App

Tracking your food intake is paramount to success when trying to burn fat. How will you know what adjustments to make if you do not remember exactly what you ate over the course of the month? You could definitely write down everything you put into your body, but then you also bear the responsibility of looking up the calories, protein, carbs, fats, etc. Not to mention the math of adding all of those up, it is exhausting just thinking about it! Instead, download an app on your phone, which you probably carry most of the time. Once you have a good library of foods built up in the database, tracking becomes a seamless. Simply enter them in and the app does all of the counting. Apps such as MyFitnessPal also allow you to form groups of friends and send messages, creating a community of people who share similar goals as yourself.

Stay Away From Artificial Sweeteners

This is easier said than done, as artificial sweeteners are becoming increasingly common in "diet" and "zero calorie" foods. Eliminating these from your diet altogether will be majorly beneficial to your health. Aside from the fact that they have been linked to certain cancers, studies have shown that these low cal sweeteners fool your brain into craving sugar, sending you searching for the sweets that can really derail your progress. Keep the fake sugars such as aspartame, saccharin, and sucralose out of the equation, and save the real sweets for a well deserved "cheat day."s

Keep Bad Foods Out of the House

How many times have you been sitting on your couch, and all of a sudden crave a bag of potato chips or ice cream? If you only have to walk to the kitchen to grab it, it does not seem like such a daunting task, and you probably end up giving in to that craving. However, if you have to get dressed, get in your car, drive to the grocery store, wait in line, pay, drive home, and THEN get to indulge in your craving, it might not seem worth it. Keep the fridge stocked with healthy snacks like fruit, veggies, cheeses, nuts, and other plant based, nutrient rich foods that will satisfy your salty or sweet tooth.

__Blend Your Vegetables__

If you are getting six to ten servings of veggies each day consistently, then you are doing better than 99% of the population. Keep it up! However, if you consistently fall short of this number, then chances are you need to try a new method of getting in those daily greens. Maybe it is because you do not like the taste, or maybe you don't like to cook them. Whatever it is, it can be fixed by the convenience of blending (or juicing) your veggies and fruits. Blending keeps the fiber, so I recommend that, but juicing is better than nothing. It only takes a little fruit to make a whole lot of veggies taste palatable. Blending with organic fruit juice or coconut water can make it even sweeter. Be careful how much of these fluids you use. They do contain sugar (although it is fructose from the fruit, make sure to get "no sugar added"). Using half water will help take the overall calories and sugar content down. Give it a try! Use a few different greens, a carrot, and a handful of blueberries with eight ounces of organic apple juice and eight ounces of water.

Supplement Wisely

There are many supplements out there that are designed to help you in your fat burning efforts. Some work great, and some not so much. Do your research on a product before you purchase it, and find a product that will work effectively for you. Choose a reputable brand, as supplements are NOT regulated by the Food and Drug Administration (FDA), and therefore, require little-to-no standards as to what is actually in the package. Also, err on the side of caution when it comes to product safety, if you are unsure about it, do not use it. Period.

Drink Green Tea

Some have called it the healthiest beverage on the planet. It is a fairly accurate statement, as green tea has various health benefits, including fat burning and improving brain function. The polyphenols found in green tea are also powerful antioxidants that help fight cancer. Additionally, it has natural caffeine in it, making it a great morning substitute for energy drinks and coffee. Squeeze a little lemon in there for taste and drink up!

Eat Spicy Food

Many different types of spices have been found to have a fat burning effect in the human body. This could be due to the increase in heat they create during the digestion process; therefore, increasing your overall calorie expenditure. Some common spices that you probably have already lying around in your kitchen include garlic, cinnamon, turmeric, chilies, cayenne pepper, ginger, mustard, and peppermint. Throw these spices into your normal recipes to add a little fat burning kick.

Consume a Slow Digesting Protein Source Before Bed

We talked about protein as a great fat burning macronutrient, and ingesting a high quality source before going to bed can help increase the amount of fat you burn during the night. It will help keep your metabolism high while you sleep, as your body breaks down the foods that you just ate. It also shortens the duration of the "fast" that often slows down the metabolism between dinner and breakfast. High quality, slow digesting sources include cottage cheese, casein protein, and lean red meats.

Drink More Water

       The recommended daily water intake is sixty-four ounces per day. New research shows that it is closer to 100 ounces for men and 72 ounces for women. However, these numbers are far too low if you are active or working out, or if you are trying to lose weight. Your body needs water to assist with brain and kidney functions, digestion, and many others. If you are even slightly dehydrated, these functions become impaired. When trying to lose fat, you need ALL of your body's systems to be working optimally in order to get the best results. To make sure you are getting enough water each day, have a couple of water bottles filled up and ready to go with you throughout the day. Make sure to drink at least 8-16 ounces with each meal and 8-16 ounces between meals. Always aim HIGHER than the recommended daily amount, there is no penalty for going over! Water is calorie free, and can also prevent hunger pangs, as it takes up space in your stomach, making you feel fuller longer.

Jumpstart With a Cleanse

Cleansing offers many health benefits, ranging from weight loss to better skin health to elimination of toxins from your digestive tract. There are not only endless benefits, but endless variations of cleansing as well. Some cleanses are strictly juice and water, while others allow small amounts of whole foods. The best one to choose is the one that you can complete ALL THE WAY THROUGH! It does not do you much good to make it half way through a Lemonade Diet and then give up. It does not work that way. If you have never tried a cleanse before, start with something short that does not completely consume your life. This will give you a better chance of making it all the way to the finish line and getting that jump start to weight loss that you are looking for.

Ditch the Food Pyramid

Whoever decided that the food pyramid was the definitive guide to eating healthy in the 21st century was mistaken. The pyramid has been used as a guideline since 1992, right around the time of the "low fat" craze that was sweeping the country. It was based on a system created twenty years prior to that by a group of Swedish scientists who were given the responsibility of creating a way of eating nutritious foods that were cost effective. Thus, eleven servings a day of grains were placed as the primary source of consumption on the bottom of the pyramid. Today, we know that amount to be counterproductive to fat loss and overall health. However, the guidelines have really not changed much over the years, despite increasing research showing that the food pyramid is in fact out dated. Do not stick with the outdated food pyramid as your guide to healthy eating, instead get your hands on the newest and most relevant dietary information (like the info found in this book!) and use it to transform your body into the one you have always wanted!

We hope that you enjoyed this book and found the tips included to be useful for your everyday routines. If possible, use the advice that we gave at the beginning of the book and try to implement and master a new strategy every week. Remember that changing your lifestyle to enable you to lose body fat is a process, not an overnight sensation. Every step you take in the right direction will get you closer to your overall goal of a leaner, healthier you. Good luck on your journey and be sure to enjoy the process of becoming a healthier version of yourself!

www.ingramcontent.com/pod-product-compliance
Lightning Source LLC
Chambersburg PA
CBHW070614290526
45790CB00002B/915